I0695565

Table of Contents

Dehydration occurs when more water and fluids leave the body than enter it. Even low levels of dehydration can cause headaches, lethargy, and constipation.

The human body is roughly 75 percent water. Without this water, it cannot survive. Water is found inside cells, within blood vessels, and between cells.

A sophisticated water management system keeps our water levels balanced, and our thirst mechanism tells us when we need to increase fluid intake.

Although water is constantly lost throughout the day as we breathe, sweat, urinate, and defecate, we can replenish the water in our body by drinking fluids. The body can also move water around to areas where it is needed most if dehydration begins to occur.

Most occurrences of dehydration can be easily reversed by increasing fluid intake, but severe cases of dehydration require immediate medical attention.

BREAKFAST

1. Spicy Vegan Burritos

Prep Time: 20 Minutes

Cook Time: 30 Minutes

Servings: 4

Ingredients

For the Roasted Potatoes:

- 1 medium russet potato, scrubbed and cut into ½ to 1 inch cubes
- 2 teaspoons olive oil
- 1 ½ teaspoons cornstarch
- 1 teaspoon ground cumin
- ¼ teaspoon onion powder
- ¼ teaspoon garlic powder
- ¼ teaspoon salt, or to taste
- For the Tofu Filling:
- 1 tablespoon olive oil
- 1 small onion, diced
- 2 garlic cloves, minced
- 7 ounces extra-firm tofu (half of a 14 ounce package)

- 1 cup canned black beans, drained and rinsed
- 1 teaspoon ground cumin
- ½ teaspoon turmeric
- ½ cup jarred salsa
- ¼ cup chopped fresh cilantro
- Salt & pepper, to taste

For the Burritos:

- 4 large (burrito sized) flour tortillas
- 1 ripe avocado, sliced
- Additional fillings of choice, such as vegan cheese, sour cream, hot sauce, and additional salsa

Instructions

Make the Potatoes

1. Preheat the oven to 400°F and line a baking sheet with parchment paper.
2. Place the potatoes into a large bowl and add the oil, cornstarch, cumin, onion powder, garlic powder, and salt.
3. Roast the potatoes for about 20 minutes, until easily pierced with a fork.

Make the Tofu Filling

1. While the potatoes roast, heat the oil in a large skillet over medium heat.

2. Add the onion and cook it for about 5 minutes, stirring frequently, until soft and translucent.

3. Stir in the garlic and sauté it with the onion for about 1 minute, until very fragrant.

4. Crumble the tofu into the skillet, then add the beans, cumin, and turmeric. Cook everything for about 2 minutes, stirring frequently, until the mixture begins to dry up.

5. Stir in the salsa and continue cooking the mixture for 5 minutes, stirring occasionally.

6. Remove the skillet from heat. Stir in the cilantro, salt and pepper.

7. Assemble the Burritos

8. Lay a tortilla on a work surface and arrange one fourth of the potatoes and one fourth of the tofu filling in a strip near the center. Add avocado slices and any other fillings you'd like to include.

9. Fold the side of the tortilla closest to you over the fillings, tuck the sides in, then roll the burrito closed.

10. Repeat until the remaining tortillas and fillings are used.

11. Serve.

Prep Time: 20 Minutes

Cook Time: 15 Minutes

Servings: 6

Ingredients

For the Spicy Cashew Cheese:

- 1 cup raw cashews, soaked in water 4 to 8 hours, drained and rinsed
- 2 tablespoons vinegar-based hot sauce (such as Cholula), plus more, to taste
- 2 tablespoons unsweetened and unflavored non-dairy milk, plus more as needed
- ½ teaspoon salt

For the Eggy Chickpea Patties:

- ⅔ cup chickpea flour
- 2 tablespoons nutritional yeast flakes
- ½ teaspoon baking powder
- ½ teaspoon ground cumin
- ½ teaspoon paprika
- ¼ teaspoon turmeric
- ¼ teaspoon Kala namak (for eggy flavor, can substitute table salt)

- ¼ teaspoon black pepper
- ½ cup water
- 1 tablespoon soy sauce
- 1 tablespoon olive oil (or high-heat oil of choice)

For the Sandwiches:

- 4 vegan English muffins, split and toasted
- ½ batch tempeh bacon (optional)
- ½ cup baby spinach
- Additional fillings or sauces of choice, such as salsa, ketchup, sliced vegan cheese, avocado, etc.

Instructions

To Make the Spicy Cashew Cheese

1. Place all ingredients into the bowl of a food processor fitted with an s-blade. Blend until smooth.
2. Taste-test the mixture and adjust the seasonings to your liking. Thin the mixture with additional milk if it seems too thick. Blend again.

To Make the Eggy Chickpea Patties

1. Whisk the chickpea flour, nutritional yeast, baking powder, cumin, paprika, turmeric, kala namak and black pepper together in a small bowl.

2. Whisk in the water and soy sauce.

3. Coat the bottom of a medium skillet with olive oil and place it over medium heat.

4. Give the oil a minute to heat up, then pour about ¼ cup of batter into the skillet, making an approximately 3-inch patty. Repeat for as many patties as you can fit into the skillet without crowding.

5. Cook the patties for 3 to 4 minutes, until bubbles form in the center, then flip and cook about 3 to 4 minutes more, until set and lightly browned.

6. Remove the patties from the skillet and transfer them to a plate. Repeat the process until all of the batter is used.

To Assemble the Sandwiches

1. Slather the inside of one or both halves of each muffin with the spicy cashew cheese, then layer and stuff with the eggy patties, tempeh bacon (if using), and spinach on the bottom halves, along with any additional fillings you choose.

2. Serve.

Prep Time: 10 Minutes

Cook Time: 40 Minutes

Servings: 4

Ingredients

- 1 ¼ cups vital wheat gluten
- ¼ cup nutritional yeast flakes
- 2 teaspoons smoked paprika
- 2 teaspoons ground black pepper
- 1 teaspoon onion powder
- ½ teaspoon dried thyme
- ¾ cup cooked brown lentils, drained
- 1 cup vegetable broth
- ¼ cup soy sauce
- 2 tablespoons maple syrup
- 2 garlic cloves, minced
- About 2 tablespoons canola oil, or high heat oil of choice

Instructions

1. Begin by setting up a steaming apparatus, such as a wok and bamboo steamer or a pot fitted with a steaming basket (see my tips above).
2. In a medium mixing bowl, stir together the wheat gluten, nutritional yeast, paprika, pepper, onion powder and thyme.
3. Stir the broth, soy sauce, maple syrup and garlic together in a separate bowl or liquid measuring cup.
4. Add the lentils to the dry mixture, then stir in the broth mixture to form a dough. Mix it up well, using your hands if needed.
5. Divide the dough in two and roll into two 6" logs. Wrap each log tightly in a sheet of parchment paper or foil and steam for 30 minutes.
6. Remove the logs from the steamer and give them a few minutes to cool.
7. Once they're cool enough to handle, remove the parchment paper or foil and slice the logs into about ½ inch thick slices (or your preferred thickness).
8. Coat the bottom of a large skillet with oil and place it over medium heat.
9. When the oil is hot, add the sausage slices and pan-fry for about 4 minutes on each side. Cook in batches if

needed. Transfer the cooked sausage patties to a paper towel-lined plate.

10. Serve.

Prep Time: 45 Minutes

Cook Time: 20 Minutes

Servings: 6

Ingredients

For the Filling:

- 2 tablespoons olive oil
- 1 medium (12 ounce) russet potato, scrubbed and diced
- 1 medium onion, diced
- 2 teaspoons ground cumin
- 1 teaspoon ground coriander seed
- 1 green bell pepper, diced
- 1 jalapeño pepper, seeded and minced (optional)
- 1 14-ounce can chickpeas, drained and rinsed
- 3 garlic cloves, minced
- 1 ripe Avocado From Mexico pitted and diced
- ¼ cup chopped fresh cilantro
- 1 tablespoon lime juice
- Salt and pepper to taste

For the Sauce:

- 1 14-ounce can tomato puree

- 3 tablespoons adobo sauce, from a can of chipotle peppers

- Salt and pepper to taste

- For Assembling the Enchiladas:

- 12 to 14 corn tortillas

For the Avocado Crema:

- 1 ripe avocado

- ½ cup unsweetened soy or almond milk

- 2 tablespoons lime juice

- Salt to taste

Instructions

1. Make the filling by coating the bottom of a large skillet with oil and placing it over medium heat. Add potato, onion, cumin and coriander. Cook for about 15 minutes, until potatoes begin to soften and brown, flipping occasionally. Add bell pepper, jalapeño, and chickpeas. Cook until bell peppers are lightly browned and potatoes are fully softened. Add garlic and cook about 1 minute more, until very fragrant. Remove from heat and add avocado, cilantro, and lime juice.

Flip gently a few times to incorporate the ingredients. Season with salt and pepper to taste.

2. Make the sauce by stirring tomato puree and adobo sauce together in a small bowl.

3. Preheat oven to 350°. Ladle about a third of the sauce into the bottom of a 9 x 13 inch baking dish (or a couple of smaller baking dishes). Lightly coat the bottom of a large skillet with oil and place it over medium heat. Place a tortilla into the skillet to warm it up, allowing it to sit in skillet for 30 seconds to 1 minute. Remove the tortilla from the skillet and place it onto a work surface. Spoon 3 to 4 tablespoons of potato mixture into the tortilla and roll. Place rolled tortilla, seam side down, into baking dish and spoon sauce over top, spreading around to coat the entire outside of the tortilla. Repeat until all tortillas are used.

4. Place the baking dish into the oven and bake until the sauce is bubbly, about 25 minutes.

5. While the enchiladas bake, place all ingredients for the avocado crema into a blender and blend until smooth and creamy. Add a splash more milk if needed.

6. When the enchiladas are done baking, divide them onto plates and top with avocado crema, along with a sprinkling of fresh cilantro, if desired. Serve.

Prep Time: 5 Minutes

Cook Time: 10 Minutes

Servings: 2

Ingredients

- 3 tablespoons soy sauce or tamari
- 1 ½ tablespoons maple syrup
- 1 tablespoons apple cider vinegar
- 1 garlic clove, minced
- 1 teaspoon smoked paprika
- ¾ teaspoon black pepper
- 1 8 ounce package tempeh
- 1 tablespoon olive oil
- 2-3 vegan English muffins, split and toasted
- ½ avocado, sliced
- About ½ cup baby spinach
- Ketchup
- Dijon mustard

Instructions

1. Whisk the soy sauce, maple syrup, vinegar, garlic, paprika and pepper together in a small bowl.

2. Slice the tempeh in half, thickness-wise, so you end up with two thin slabs. Slice each of your slabs in half or thirds, so you end up with 4-6 slabs total.

3. Coat a large skillet with olive oil and place it over medium-high heat. Add the tempeh slabs in an even layer and cook until they're browned on the bottoms, about 3 minutes. Pour soy sauce mixture over tempeh and cook another minute or so, until the sauce dries up and forms a thick coating on the tempeh.

4. Flip tempeh slabs and cook about 3 more minutes, until browned on opposite sides and most of the liquid has cooked off.

5. Slather the English muffins with ketchup, Dijon and any other dressings you like. Stuff the muffins with tempeh slabs, topped with avocado slices and baby spinach.

Prep Time: 20 Minutes

Cook Time: 18 Minutes

Servings: 12

Ingredients

- 1 small overripe banana, mashed
- ¼ cup melted coconut oil
- 2 tablespoons coconut sugar
- 1 teaspoon vanilla extract
- ¾ cup oat flour, store bought, or make it by processing rolled oats in a food processor
- ½ cup rolled oats
- ½ teaspoon baking powder
- 1 teaspoon ground cinnamon
- ½ teaspoon powdered ginger
- ¼ teaspoon salt
- ½ Granny Smith apple, shredded
- ¾ cup shredded carrots, about 2 carrots
- ¼ cup unsweetened flaked coconut
- ¼ cup chopped walnuts
- ¼ cup raisins

Instructions

1. Preheat oven to 350° and line a baking sheet with parchment paper.

2. Stir the banana, coconut oil, sugar and vanilla together in a medium bowl. In a separate medium mixing bowl, stir together the oat flour, oats, baking powder, cinnamon, ginger, and salt. Add the banana mixture to the oat mixture and stir just until fully blended. Fold in the apple, carrots, coconut, walnuts, and raisins. The batter should be moist, but you should be able to shape it into balls.

3. Shape about 3 tablespoons of the batter into a ball and place on the prepared baking sheet. Continue until all of the batter is used, making about a dozen balls and spacing them at least an inch apart.

4. Bake for about 18 minutes. I like to flatten my cookies out with the back of a spoon after about 10 minutes. The cookies will be soft, but they should hold together, and will firm up a bit as they cool.

Prep Time: 10 Minutes

Cook Time: 25 Minutes

Servings: 12

Ingredients

- 2 ½ cups all-purpose flour
- ¾ cup organic granulated sugar
- 1 tablespoon baking powder
- ½ teaspoon baking soda
- 1 teaspoon ground cinnamon
- ½ teaspoon salt
- 1 cup plus 2 tablespoons unsweetened non-dairy milk
- ½ cup canola oil, or suitable baking oil of choice
- 2 teaspoons vanilla extract
- 1 teaspoon apple cider vinegar
- 1 ½ cups vegan chocolate chips
- 1 tablespoon organic brown sugar

Instructions

1. Preheat the oven to 375°F and line a 12-cup muffin tin with paper liners.

2. In a large mixing bowl whisk together the flour, sugar, baking powder, baking soda, cinnamon, and salt.

3. In a separate container such as a liquid measuring cup, stir together the milk, oil, vanilla, and vinegar.

4. Pour the milk mixture into the bowl with the flour mixture and stir everything together just until combined.

5. Fold in the chocolate chips.

6. Divide the batter among the muffin cups, then sprinkle the tops of the unbaked muffins with brown sugar.

7. Bake the muffins for 20 to 22 minutes, until lightly browned on top and set. You can test for doneness by lightly touching a finger to the top of a muffin, then removing it. If the muffin is done it will spring back.

8. Transfer the muffin tin to a cooling rack and allow the muffins to cool (until just warm or cooler) before removing them from the tin.

Prep Time: 10 Minutes

Cook Time: 25 Minutes

Servings: 2

Ingredients

- 2 ripe peaches sliced thinly
- 3 tbsp. maple syrup divided
- 1 tsp. cinnamon
- 1 ½ cup unsweetened unflavored non-dairy milk
- 1 tsp. vanilla extract
- ½ cup polenta
- a few pecan pieces optional

Instructions

1. Preheat oven to 375. Spray baking dish or cast iron skillet with nonstick cooking spray. Add peaches, 2 tbsp. maple syrup and cinnamon. Toss to coat peaches. Bake about 20 minutes, or until tender and syrupy.
2. While your peaches bake, prepare your polenta. Start by bringing milk, vanilla and 1 tbsp. maple syrup to a simmer in medium saucepan. Add polenta. Cook

about five minutes, stirring frequently, or until thick and creamy.

3. Spoon into bowls. You can add a little extra milk and/or syrup here if you'd like it sweeter and/or creamier. Top with peaches and pecans.

Prep Time: 15 Minutes

Cook Time: 20 Minutes

Servings: 4

Ingredients

- 2 tablespoons canola oil, or high heat oil of choice
- 1 small (8 ounce/227 gram) russet potato, diced into about ½ inch pieces
- 1 medium onion, diced
- 1 bell pepper (any color), roughly chopped
- 3 garlic cloves, minced
- 1 (14 ounce/400 gram) package extra firm tofu, drained and patted dry
- 2 cups roughly chopped kale leaves
- 2 tablespoons soy sauce1
- 2 tablespoons nutritional yeast flakes
- 2 teaspoons ground cumin
- 1 teaspoon ground turmeric
- 1 tablespoon hot sauce (such as Cholula) or to taste
- Black pepper, to taste
- Kala namak, to taste (optional - for eggy flavor)
- Toppings or accompaniments of choice

Instructions

1. Coat the bottom of a large nonstick skillet with the oil and place it over medium heat.

2. Give the oil a minute to heat up, and when it begins to shimmer add the potato.

3. Cook the potato, flipping occasionally, until the pieces are just fork tender and crisp on the outside, about 8 minutes2.

4. Add the onion to the skillet and cook it with the potato until it just begins to soften, about 3 minutes, continuing to flip everything occasionally.

5. Add the bell pepper. Cook everything for about another two minutes, until the pepper begins to soften up.

6. Push everything to the sides of the skillet and add the garlic to the middle. Cook the garlic for about 1 minute, until very fragrant.

7. Break tofu into bite-sized chunks and add it to skillet. Flip everything a few times with a spatula to mix the ingredients.

8. Cook the mixture for about 5 minutes, flipping occasionally and breaking up chunks of tofu as needed, until the tofu begins to dry up and crisp in spots.

9. Add the kale, in batches if needed, letting each batch wilt slightly before adding the next.

10. Stir in the soy sauce, nutritional yeast, cumin, and turmeric. Flip everything again to incorporate the ingredients. Cook for 1 to 2 minutes, until most of the soy sauce dries up and the kale has fully wilted.

11. Remove the skillet from heat and season the scramble with hot sauce, kala namak (or table salt), and black pepper to taste.

12. Serve with toppings and accompaniments of choice.

Prep Time: 10 Minutes

Cook Time: 10 Minutes

Servings: 10

Ingredients

- 3 medium overripe bananas
- ⅓ cup organic granulated sugar
- ⅓ cup organic brown sugar
- ⅓ cup canola oil (or your favorite baking oil)
- 2 teaspoons vanilla extract
- 2 cups all-purpose flour
- 1 teaspoon baking soda
- 1 teaspoon ground cinnamon
- 1 teaspoon salt
- 1 cup chopped walnuts (or pecans, vegan chocolate chips, or your favorite banana bread stir-in)

For Topping:

- ¼ cup organic brown sugar

Instructions

1. Preheat the oven to 350°.

2. Lightly oil a 9-inch loaf pan and arrange a strip of parchment paper width-wise along the center, with just a bit hanging out over each side.

3. Peel the bananas and place them into a large mixing bowl. Mash them well with a fork or potato masher.

4. Add sugar, brown sugar, oil, and vanilla to the bowl. Stir until well-mixed.

5. Add the flour to the bowl, then sprinkle the baking soda, cinnamon and salt on top of the flour.

6. Stir everything together just until mixed. Don't overmix. The batter will be thick.

7. Fold in the walnuts.

8. Spoon the batter into the prepared loaf pan and smooth out the top with the back of a spoon.

9. Sprinkle the top with brown sugar.

10. Bake for 50 minutes, or until a toothpick inserted into the center comes out clean.

11. Remove the pan from the oven and transfer it to a wire rack. Allow the loaf to cool for at least 15 minutes before removing it from the pan.

12. Slice and serve.

11. Vegan Pepperoni

Prep Time: 10 Minutes

Cook Time: 40 Minutes

Servings: 10

Ingredients

- 1 ¼ cup vital wheat gluten
- ½ cup precooked or canned chickpeas (drain and rinse if using canned)
- 3 garlic cloves, minced
- 3 tablespoons water, plus more if needed
- ¼ cup soy sauce
- 1 tablespoon olive oil
- 2 teaspoons red wine vinegar
- 1 teaspoon maple syrup
- ½ teaspoon liquid smoke
- 1 ½ tablespoons sweet paprika
- 1 ½ teaspoons fennel seed
- 1 teaspoon onion powder
- 1 teaspoon red pepper flakes
- ½ teaspoon cayenne pepper

- ½ teaspoon black pepper

Instructions

1. Prepare your steaming device and bring your water to a boil so you're ready to start steaming as soon as the dough is mixed.
2. Place all ingredients into the bowl of a food processor fitted with an s-blade. (Note 1)
3. Turn on the machine until the mixture is fully blended.
4. Grab a small amount of the mixture and pinch it together in your hand. It should hold together like a firm dough. If it's too crumbly, add a bit more water and blend again
5. Remove the dough from the food processor and divide it into two equal portions.
6. Roll the dough portions into logs and place each on a sheet of foil. (Note 2)
7. Wrap the logs in foil, rolling and shaping as you go, so that they are each about 8-inches long when you're done. (Note 3)
8. Place the dough logs in your steamer and steam them for 40 minutes.

9. Once they're done steaming, remove the vegan pepperoni logs from the steamer and let them cool. After a few minutes you can carefully open the foil.

10. Once they are cool, place the pepperoni logs into sealed containers or bags and chill them until cold throughout, about 3 hours.

11. Thinly slice your vegan pepperoni into around 70 slices.

12. Serve or place in an airtight container and store for later.

Prep Time: 15 Minutes

Cook Time: 20 Minutes

Servings: 16

Ingredients

- 3 cups fresh corn kernels, about 4 ears worth of corn
- 1 cup all-purpose flour
- 2 tablespoons cornmeal
- ½ teaspoon baking powder
- ½ teaspoon ground cumin (optional)
- ¾ teaspoon salt
- ¾ cup unflavored and unsweetened non-dairy milk
- ½ cup peanut oil, or as needed (for fried fritters only)
- Jalapeño slices (optional)

Instructions

1. If you're planning on baking your fritters, preheat the oven to 400°F and line a couple of baking sheets with parchment paper.
2. Stir the corn, flour, cornmeal, baking powder, and salt together in a large mixing bowl.

3. Pour in the milk and stir, just until the ingredients are thoroughly mixed.

4. For Fried Fritters

5. Generously coat the bottom of a medium nonstick skillet with the oil (about ⅛ inch deep) and place it over medium heat.

6. Once the oil begins to shimmer, drop the batter into the skillet, using about ⅓ cup for each fritter. Optionally place a jalapeño slice or two on top of each fritter. Cook the fritters in batches, frying as many as you can at a time without crowding the skillet.

7. Cook the fritters for 3 to 4 minutes on each side, carefully testing each one before flipping to make sure it's ready and will hold together.

8. Transfer the cooked fritters to a paper towel-lined plate to drain while you cook the remaining ones, adding oil to the skillet as needed between batches.

9. Serve.

For Baked Fritters

1. Drop the batter by ⅓ cupfuls on the prepared baking sheets. Optionally place a jalapeño slice or two on top of each fritter.

2. Bake the fritters until they appear solid, about 12 to 15 minutes. They will only darken slightly since they're being cooked without oil.

3. Remove the baking sheets from the oven and place them on a cooling rack. Let the fritters cool for a few minutes before removing them from the baking sheets.

4. Serve.

Prep Time: 15 Minutes

Cook Time: 25 Minutes

Servings: 4

Ingredients

- o ounces dried ramen noodles (half of a 9.5 ounce package)
- 2 tablespoons peanut oil, divided
- 8 ounces super firm tofu, drained and cut into ½ inch cubes
- 1 small onion, thinly sliced into half rings
- 3 garlic cloves, minced
- 2 cups vegan kimchi, roughly chopped, solids and juice separated
- 5 cups vegetable broth
- 1 tablespoon gochujang, plus more to taste
- 1 teaspoon toasted sesame oil
- ½ cup frozen shelled edamame, thawed
- 2 scallions, chopped
- Toasted sesame seeds

Instructions

1. Bring a large pot of water to boil and cook the noodles according to the package directions. Drain them into a colander when done.
2. While the noodles cook, coat the bottom of a large skillet with 1 tablespoon of the peanut oil and place it over medium heat.
3. Once the oil is hot, add the tofu cubes in an even layer. Cook the tofu for about 10 minutes, flipping the pieces once or twice so they brown on multiple sides. Transfer the cooked tofu to a plate when done.
4. While the tofu cooks, coat the bottom of a large pot with the remaining oil and place it over medium heat.
5. Once the oil is hot add the onion. Sweat the onion for about 5 minutes, until soft and translucent.
6. Add the garlic to the pot and cook it with the onion for about 1 minute, until very fragrant.
7. Add the kimchi solids to the pot, reserving the juice. Sauté the kimchi for about 2 minutes, stirring frequently.
8. Stir in the broth and gochujang.
9. Raise the heat and bring the soup to a boil. Lower the heat and allow it to simmer for about 10 minutes, until the kimchi is very soft.

10. Remove the pot from heat and stir in the sesame oil. Season the soup with salt if desired.

11. Divide the noodles, edamame, and cooked tofu among four bowls, then ladle the broth over everything. Sprinkle with scallions and sesame seeds.

12. Serve.

Prep Time: 20 Minutes

Cook Time: 5 Minutes

Servings: 5

Ingredients

- 1 (9.5 ounce or 269 gram) package soba noodles
- ½ cup creamy natural peanut butter
- 5 tablespoons soy sauce, plus more to taste
- 4 tablespoons lime juice, plus more to taste
- 4 tablespoons maple syrup, plus more to taste
- 1 garlic clove, minced
- 1 teaspoon freshly grated ginger
- ¼ cup water, plus more as needed
- 1 medium red bell pepper, sliced into strips
- 2 cups shredded red cabbage
- 2 medium carrots, julienne cut
- 1 cup frozen shelled edamame, thawed
- 2 scallions, sliced
- ¼ cup chopped fresh basil
- ¼ cup chopped fresh cilantro
- Toasted sesame seeds

Instructions

1. Bring a large pot of water to a boil. Add the soba noodles and cook them according to the package directions.
2. Drain the noodles into a colander and rinse them with cold water until completely cool. Let them sit in the colander for a few minutes to allow any excess water to drain.
3. While the noodles cook, make the dressing. Whisk the peanut butter, soy sauce, lime juice, maple syrup, garlic and ginger together in a small bowl. Thin with water as needed until the dressing is creamy but pourable.
4. Place the noodles into a large mixing bowl with the pepper, cabbage, carrots, edamame, scallions, basil, and cilantro.
5. Pour the dressing into the bowl and toss the mixture to coat everything with dressing.
6. Taste-test the salad and add more soy sauce, lime juice and/or maple syrup to taste.
7. Divide onto plates and top each with sesame seeds.
8. Serve.

Prep Time: 10 Minutes

Cook Time: 25 Minutes

Servings: 12

Ingredients

For the Chipotle Mayo:

- ½ cup vegan mayo
- 1 teaspoon vinegar-based hot sauce (such as Cholula)
- ½ teaspoon chipotle chile powder
- ½ teaspoon smoked paprika
- Salt to taste

For the Vegetable Fritters:

- ½ pound carrots (about 2 to 3 medium carrots) shredded
- ½ pound broccoli (about 1 small crown), finely minced
- ¼ cup chopped scallions (about 2 scallions)
- 1 garlic clove, minced
- ⅔ cup all-purpose flour
- ⅓ cup panko breadcrumbs
- ½ teaspoon ground cumin

- Pinch cayenne pepper

- 1 teaspoon salt

- ½ teaspoon black pepper

- ½ cup water

- 1 tablespoon lemon juice

- ⅓ cup peanut oil (or high heat oil of choice), plus more as needed

For Serving:

- Chopped chives (optional)

Instructions

1. Begin my making the chipotle mayo. Mix all ingredients in a small bowl. Taste-test and adjust the seasonings to your liking.

2. To make the fritters, add the carrots, broccoli, scallions, and garlic to a large mixing bowl. Stir to evenly distribute the ingredients.

3. Add the flour, breadcrumbs, cumin, cayenne pepper, salt, and black pepper. Stir until well-mixed.

4. Stir in the lemon juice and water. Test the mixture by pressing some together in your hands. It should hold

together. If the mixture is too crumbly, add a splash of water. If it's too wet, add a bit of flour.

5. Place a medium skillet over medium heat. Add oil to the skillet until it's about ⅛ inch deep.

6. When the oil begins to shimmer, shape the veggie mixture into 2-inch patties and add them directly to the skillet. Only add as many patties as you can fit without crowding the skillet.

7. Cook the fritters for about 4 minutes on each side, until browned and crispy. Transfer the cooked fritters to a paper towel-lined plate.

8. Continue cooking the fritters in batches until all of the veggie mixture has been used. Add oil to the skillet between batches as needed.

9. Serve the fritters with a sprinkling of chives (optional) with aioli on the side.

Prep Time: 10 Minutes

Cook Time: 35 Minutes

Servings: 6

Ingredients

- 1 tablespoon canola oil
- 1 medium onion, diced
- 4 garlic cloves, minced
- 2 teaspoons freshly grated ginger
- 2 teaspoons garam masala
- 1 teaspoon cumin seeds
- ½ teaspoon ground turmeric
- Pinch cayenne pepper, optional (or to taste)
- 2 cups dried split red lentils
- 6 cups vegetable broth
- 1 cup full-fat coconut milk
- 1 (14 ounce or 400 gram) can diced tomatoes
- 2 tablespoons lemon juice
- Salt & pepper, to taste
- Chopped fresh cilantro, for topping

Instructions

1. Coat the bottom of a large pot with oil and place it over medium heat.

2. Give the oil a minute to heat up, the add the onion. Sweat the onion for about 5 minutes, until it becomes soft and translucent.

3. Stir in the garlic, ginger, garam masala, cumin seeds, turmeric, and cayenne pepper. Cook everything for about 1 minute, until the mixture becomes very fragrant.

4. Stir in the lentils and broth. Raise the heat and bring the mixture to a boil.

5. Lower the heat and allow the soup to simmer, uncovered, for about 20 minutes, until the lentils are very soft.

6. Stir in the coconut milk and tomatoes. Continue simmering for about 5 minutes, until the soup is very thick and the lentils have fallen apart.

7. Remove the pot from the burner and stir in the lemon juice. Season the soup with salt and pepper to taste.

8. Ladle into bowls and top with fresh cilantro. Serve.

Prep Time: 10 Minutes

Cook Time: 10 Minutes

Servings: 4

Ingredients

- 1 ½ teaspoons olive oil
- 8 ounces extra-firm or super firm tofu (pressed if using extra-firm), cut-into ½-inch cubes
- 2 tablespoons balsamic vinegar
- 1 teaspoon organic brown sugar
- Salt & pepper, to taste
- 4 large (10-inch) flour tortillas or wraps
- ½ cup hummus
- ½ cup baby spinach leaves
- 1 medium tomato, thinly sliced
- ½ ripe avocado, pitted, peeled, and sliced
- 8-12 large fresh basil leaves
- ½ medium cucumber, julienne cut

Instructions

1. Coat the bottom of a large skillet with the oil and place it over medium heat.

2. Give the oil a minute to heat up, then add the tofu cubes.

3. Cook the tofu for about 10 minutes, flipping the pieces once or twice, until browned on multiple sides.

4. While the tofu cooks, stir the balsamic vinegar and brown sugar together in a small bowl.

5. When the tofu has finished cooking, carefully pour the balsamic mixture over the pieces. Flip them a few times and continue cooking them for about 2 minutes, until all of the liquid cooks off.

6. Remove the tofu from the skillet and season the pieces with salt to taste.

7. Spread about 2 tablespoons of hummus in a short strip down the middle of each tortilla, then arrange the fillings over the hummus in the following order: spinach, tomato, avocado, basil, cucumber, and tofu, sprinkling the layers lightly with salt and pepper to taste as you arrange.

8. Fold the edge of one of the wraps over the fillings, then tuck in the sides and roll the wrap to close. Repeat for each wrap.

9. Optionally slice the wraps in half. Serve.

Prep Time: 10 Minutes

Cook Time: 8 Minutes

Servings: 4

Ingredients

- 1 cup cooked or canned chickpeas, drained and rinsed
- 1 (14 ounce or 400 gram) can or jar heart of palm, roughly chopped (¼ to ½ inch chunks)
- 1 medium celery stalk, diced
- 2 tablespoons vegan mayonnaise
- 1 tablespoon lemon juice
- 2 tablespoons chopped fresh chives
- 1 tablespoon chopped fresh dill
- 1 teaspoon Old Bay seasoning
- ½ teaspoon sweet paprika, plus more for topping
- Salt & pepper, to taste
- 4 hot dog rolls
- 2 tablespoons vegan butter, melted

Instructions

1. Place the chickpeas into a large mixing bowl and roughly mash them with a fork or potato masher. You want about half of them to be smashed.

2. Add the heart of palm, celery, mayonnaise, lemon juice, chives, dill, Old Bay, and paprika. Gently stir the mixture until the ingredients are evenly distributed.

3. Taste-test the mixture and season it with salt and pepper to taste. Adjust any other seasonings to your taste.

4. Place a medium skillet or grill pan on the stove over medium heat.

5. Brush the sides of one of the hot dog rolls with butter, covering the entire outer surface with a thin coating, then place the roll in the skillet. Repeat and add another roll (or as many as you can fit in a batch).

6. Toast the hot dog rolls in batches, toasting each roll for 1 to 2 minutes per side.

7. Stuff the filling into the buns and serve.

Prep Time: 10 Minutes

Cook Time: 20 Minutes

Servings: 6

Ingredients

- 1 cup uncooked quinoa
- 1 ¾ cups water
- ¼ cup olive oil
- 2 tablespoons freshly squeezed lemon juice
- 2 tablespoons red wine vinegar
- 1 large garlic clove, minced
- ½ teaspoon salt, plus more to taste (I used ¾ teaspoon)
- 2 cups diced cucumber (about 1 medium cucumber)
- 1 cup diced tomato (about 1 medium tomato)
- 1 cup cooked or canned chickpeas, drained and rinsed
- ½ cup pitted Kalamata olives, halved
- ½ cup chopped scallions (about 3 scallions)
- ¼ cup finely chopped fresh parsley, lightly packed
- ¼ cup finely chopped fresh mint, lightly packed
- Black pepper, to taste

Instructions

1. Rinse the quinoa well under cold running water (you can skip this if the package tells you it's already rinsed).

2. Stir the quinoa and water together in a small saucepan, then place it over high heat.

3. Bring the water to a boil. Lower the heat and cover. Allow the quinoa to simmer, covered, until all of the water is absorbed, about 20 minutes.

4. Remove the pot from heat and allow to sit, covered, for 5 minutes.

5. Transfer the cooked quinoa to a medium bowl and allow it to cool completely.

6. To make the dressing, stir the olive oil, lemon juice, vinegar, garlic, and ½ teaspoon of salt together in a small bowl or liquid measuring cup.

7. Add the cucumber, tomatoes, chickpeas, olives, scallions, parsley, and mint to the bowl with the quinoa.

8. Pour the dressing over the ingredients in the bowl, then stir until the ingredients are evenly mixed and coated with the dressing.

9. Season the salad with additional salt and pepper to taste.

10. Serve immediately or chill for later.

Prep Time: 15 Minutes

Cook Time: 05 Minutes

Servings: 8

Ingredients

- 3 medium ears fresh corn, shucked
- ¼ cup lime juice
- ¼ cup olive oil
- 1 garlic clove, minced
- 1 teaspoon ground cumin
- ½ teaspoon salt, plus more to taste
- 2 medium just ripe avocados, diced
- 2 cups cherry tomatoes, halved
- ¼ cup diced red onion
- ¼ cup chopped fresh cilantro

Instructions

1. Bring a large pot of water to a boil. Add the corn (still on the cobs) and boil it for 3 minutes.
2. While the corn boils, fill a large bowl or pot with ice water.

3. After the corn has finished boiling, remove the pot from heat, then use tongs to remove the cobs and transfer them directly to the ice water bath. Let the corn sit in the bath for a minute or two, until cool, before removing it from the ice bath.

4. Use a sharp knife to cut the corn kernels from each cob.

5. Make the dressing by mixing the lime juice, olive oil, garlic, cumin and salt in a small container.

6. Place the corn kernels into a large mixing bowl. Add the avocado, cherry tomatoes, onion, and cilantro.

7. Pour the dressing over the corn mixture and stir to distribute the ingredients.

8. Taste-test the salad and season it with additional salt to taste. Adjust any other seasonings to your liking.

9. Serve.

21. Vegan "Chicken" & Rice Soup

Prep Time: 15 Minutes

Cook Time: 1hrs 15 Minutes

Servings: 6

Ingredients

- 1 tablespoon olive oil
- 1 medium onion, diced
- 2 medium carrots, sliced
- 2 medium celery stalks, diced
- 1 (8 ounce or 226 gram) package seitan, finely diced
- 3 garlic cloves, minced
- 6 cups vegetable broth (plus up to 2 additional cups, as needed)
- 1 teaspoon dried thyme
- ½ teaspoon rubbed sage
- 1 bay leaf
- 1 cup dried long grain brown rice
- 1 teaspoon white wine vinegar
- Salt and pepper, to taste

Instructions

1. Coat the bottom of a large pot with the oil and place it over medium heat.
2. When the oil is hot, add the onion, carrots and celery. Cook the veggies for about 5 minutes, stirring frequently, until they begin to soften.
3. Add the seitan to the pot and cook it with the veggies for about 5 minutes, until it begins to brown.
4. Add the garlic to the pot and cook everything for about a minute, until the garlic becomes very fragrant.
5. Stir in 6 cups of broth, thyme, sage, bay leaf and rice. Raise the heat and bring the broth to a boil.
6. Lower the heat and allow the soup to simmer until the rice is tender, about 50 minutes, stirring frequently. Add up to 2 cups of additional broth if it reduces too much during cooking.
7. Remove the pot from heat and stir in the vinegar. Remove the bay leaf. Season the soup with salt and pepper to taste.
8. Ladle into bowls and serve.

Prep Time: 15 Minutes

Cook Time: 15 Minutes

Servings: 1

Ingredients

- 1 tablespoon olive oil
- 4 ounces sliced cremini mushrooms (about 2 cups of mushrooms)
- 1 garlic clove, minced
- 2 tablespoons dry white wine
- 2 tablespoons sliced fresh sage
- Salt and pepper, to taste
- 1 or 2 slices bread, toasted (I like sourdough or multigrain for this recipe)

Instructions

1. Coat the bottom of a medium skillet with the oil and place it over medium heat.
2. Once the oil is hot, add the mushrooms in an even layer. Sprinkle them with a pinch of salt.

3. Let the mushrooms cook, undisturbed, for about 5 minutes, flip and cook them for 5 minutes more, until tender and browned on both sides.

4. Push the mushrooms to the side of the skillet. If the skillet seems dry at this point, add an extra dash of oil, then add the garlic.

5. Cook the garlic for about 1 minute, stirring frequently, until very fragrant.

6. Stir in the wine, bring it to a simmer, and continue cooking everything until most of the liquid has evaporated, 2 or 3 minutes.

7. Remove the skillet from heat and stir in the sage. Season the mushrooms with salt and pepper to taste.

8. Spoon the mushrooms over the toast. Serve.

Prep Time: 15 Minutes

Cook Time: 20 Minutes

Servings: 4

Ingredients

- 7 ounces dried spaghetti (or noodles of choice)
- For the Peanut Sesame Sauce
- ⅓ cup creamy natural peanut butter
- ¼ cup soy sauce or tamari
- 2 tablespoons rice vinegar
- 2 tablespoons maple syrup
- 1 tablespoon toasted sesame oil
- About ⅓ cup water, or as needed

For the Pan-Fried Tofu:

- 1 tablespoon peanut oil, or high heat oil of choice
- 7 ounces super firm tofu, cut into 1-inch cubes

For the Peanut Noodles:

- 1 tablespoon peanut oil, or high heat oil of choice
- 3 garlic cloves, minced
- 2 teaspoons freshly grated ginger

- 4 scallions, white and green parts separated and chopped
- 2 cups shredded red cabbage

For Serving:

- ¼ cup chopped roasted peanuts
- 2 tablespoons toasted sesame seeds

Instructions

1. Bring a large pot of salted water to a boil. Add the pasta and cook it according to the package directions.
2. While the pasta cooks, whisk the ingredients for the peanut sesame sauce together in a small bowl, thinning the mixture with as much water as you need. You want the sauce to be thick and creamy, but pourable and not too runny.
3. Drain the pasta into a colander and return it to the pot.
4. Next, make the pan-fried tofu. Coat the bottom of a large skillet with 1 tablespoon of peanut oil and place it over medium heat.
5. When the oil is hot, add the tofu in an even layer. Cook the pieces for about 10 minutes, flipping one or

two times, until the cubes are browned and crispy on multiple sides.

6. Remove the tofu from the skillet and transfer it to a plate when done.

7. Add a tablespoon of peanut oil to the skillet, then add the garlic, ginger and white parts of scallions. Sauté the aromatics for about 1 minute, until very fragrant.

8. Add the noodles and tofu sauce the skillet, then the sauce. Stir everything with a fork to coat the noodles and tofu with the sauce. Raise the heat to high and cook everything for about a minute, just until heated throughout.

9. Remove the skillet from heat and stir in the cabbage.

10. Top the noodles with the peanuts, sesame seeds, and green parts of scallions. Divide onto plates and serve.

Prep Time: 20 Minutes

Cook Time: 20 Minutes

Servings: 4

Ingredients

- 1 pound butternut squash, peeled and diced (½ inch)
- 1 medium onion, peeled, quartered and layers separated
- 4 garlic cloves, peeled
- 1 tablespoon olive oil
- 12 ounces dried fettuccine pasta
- 1 cup unflavored and unsweetened non-dairy milk
- ½ cup full-fat coconut milk
- 1 teaspoon salt, plus more to taste
- ⅛ teaspoon ground nutmeg
- Black pepper, to taste
- 1 tablespoon fresh sage leaves, finely chopped

Instructions

1. Preheat the oven to 400°F.

2. Place the squash, onion, and garlic cloves on a baking sheet and drizzle them with the oil. Use your hands to rub the oil all over the veggies.

3. Place the baking sheet into the oven and roast the vegetables for about 20 minutes, until the squash is tender. Keep an eye on everything and remove any onion pieces if they begin to burn.

4. While the veggies roast, bring a large pot of salted water to a boil. Add the pasta and cook it according to the package directions.

5. Drain the pasta into a colander, reserving about ½ cup of the water that you boiled it in. Return the drained pasta to the pot.

6. When the vegetables are finished roasting place them into a blender or the bowl of a food processor fitted with an s-blade. Add the milk, coconut milk, salt, and nutmeg.

7. Blend everything until smooth.

8. Taste-test the sauce and add more salt if desired, as well as some black pepper to taste.

9. Pour the sauce over the pasta and add the sage. Stir everything up with a fork and thin the sauce with some of the reserved pasta water if needed.

10. Season the pasta with additional salt and pepper to taste, if desired.

11. Serve.

25. Vegan Goulash

Prep Time: 15 Minutes

Cook Time: 40 Minutes

Servings: 6

Ingredients

- ¾ cup dried brown lentils
- 2 tablespoons olive oil
- 6 ounces cremini mushrooms, cleaned and roughly chopped
- 1 onion, diced
- 1 red bell pepper, diced
- 3 garlic cloves, minced
- 3 cups vegetable broth
- 1 (14 ounce or 400 gram) can tomato sauce
- 1 (14 ounce or 400 gram) can diced tomatoes
- 1 teaspooon sweet paprika
- ½ teaspoon smoked papkria (can sub more sweet paprika)
- ½ teaspoon dried thyme
- ½ teaspoon dried oregano
- 2 tablespoons soy sauce
- 2 bay leaves

- 8 ounces uncooked elbow macaroni pasta (2 cups of of uncooked pasta)
- ¼ cup tomato paste
- Salt and pepper, to taste

For Serving:

- Cashew sour cream, or unflavored vegan yogurt
- Fresh parsley

Instructions

1. Place the lentils into a small saucepan and cover them with a couple of inches of water.
2. Place the pot over high heat and bring the water to a boil. Lower the heat and simmer the lentils, uncovered until they're tender but not mushy, about 25 to 30 minutes. Add water to the pot if it dries up while simmering.
3. Drain the lentils into a colander and set them aside.
4. While the lentils cook, coat the bottom of a large pot with olive oil and place it over medium heat. When the oil is hot, add the mushrooms.
5. Cook the mushrooms, flipping them once or twice, for about 5 minutes, until they begin to soften and brown.

6. Add the onion to the pot and cook it with the mushrooms for about 5 minutes more, until the onion is soft and translucent.

7. Add the bell pepper and garlic to the pot. Continue to sauté the mixture until the garlic becomes very fragrant, about 1 minute.

8. Stir in the broth, tomato sauce, tomatoes, sweet paprika, smoked paprika, thyme, oregano, soy sauce, bay leaves, and pasta. Raise heat and bring the mixture to a boil. Lower heat and allow everything to simmer until the pasta is al dente, about 20 minutes, stirring occasionally.

9. Stir in the lentils and tomato paste and allow everything to cook for about 2 more minutes, just to heat everything throughout and thicken the sauce.

10. Remove the pot from heat. Remove the bay leaves and season the goulash with salt and pepper to taste.

11. Serve with vegan yogurt, cashew cream, and/or fresh parsley.

Prep Time: 15 Minutes

Cook Time: 45 Minutes

Servings: 6

Ingredients

- ¼ cup vegan butter
- 1 large onion, diced
- 1 cup diced celery (about 3 stalks)
- 1 cup chopped carrots (about 3 carrots)
- 4 garlic cloves, minced
- 3 tablespoons all-purpose flour
- 2 ½ cup vegetable broth
- 2 ½ cups unflavored non-dairy milk
- 1 ¾ pounds Russet potatoes (about 4 medium potatoes), scrubbed, peeled, and cut into 1-inch pieces
- 1 teaspoon dried thyme
- 2 bay leaves
- 1 ½ teaspoons white wine vinegar
- Salt and pepper to taste

Instructions

1. Melt the butter in a large pot over medium heat.

2. Add the onion, celery, and carrot. Sweat the veggies until softened, about 10 minutes, stirring frequently.

3. Add the garlic to the pot and cook it for about 1 minute, until very fragrant.

4. Begin sprinkling the flour into the pot, a bit at a time, stirring between additions so the flour coats the veggies. Cook the veggies and flour for about a minute, stirring frequently.

5. Begin adding broth to the pot, a bit at a time, whisking each addition in to eliminate any lumps formed by the flour.

6. Once all the broth has been added, stir in the milk, potatoes, bay leaf and thyme.

7. Raise the heat and bring the liquid to a boil.

8. Lower the heat and allow the soup to simmer, stirring occasionally, until the base thickens a bit and the potatoes are tender, about 25 to 30 minutes.

9. Remove the pot from heat. Remove and discard the bay leaves. Stir in the vinegar and season the soup with salt and pepper to taste.

10. Ladle into bowls and serve.

Prep Time: 15 Minutes

Cook Time: 20 Minutes

Servings: 4

Ingredients

- 1 tablespoon canola oil

- 1 medium onion, diced

- 3 garlic cloves, minced

- 2 teaspoons freshly grated ginger

- 1 teaspoon whole cumin seeds

- 1 teaspoon garam masala

- ½ teaspoon ground turmeric

- 1 (15 ounce or 400 gram) can chickpeas, drained and rinsed

- 1 cup canned diced tomatoes in juice

- ¾ cup full fat coconut milk (from a can)

- 1 (10 ounce or 283 gram) package chopped frozen spinach, thawed and squeezed to remove excess water

- ½ teaspoon salt, or to taste

- Black pepper, to taste

- Chopped fresh cilantro, for serving (optional)

- Cooked basmati rice or naan, for serving

Instructions

1. Coat the bottom of a medium skillet with the oil and place it over medium heat.

2. Once the oil is hot, add the onion. Sweat the onion for about 5 minutes, stirring frequently, until it becomes soft and translucent.

3. Stir in the garlic, ginger, cumin, garam masala, and turmeric. Cook the mixture for about 1 minute, stirring constantly, until it becomes very fragrant.

4. Stir in the chickpeas, tomatoes and coconut milk. Raise the heat and bring the sauce to a simmer. Lower the heat and allow the mixture to cook for 8 to 10 minutes, stirring occasionally, until thickened slightly.

5. Stir in the spinach and let the mixture simmer for about 5 minutes more, stirring occasionally.

6. Remove the skillet from heat and season the curry with salt and pepper.

7. Serve (optionally) with a sprinkle of cilantro and basmati rice or naan.

Prep Time: 15 Minutes

Cook Time: 25 Minutes

Servings: 4

Ingredients

- 8 ounces dried rigatoni pasta
- 3 tablespoons olive oil, plus more if needed, divided
- 1 medium (1 pound or 450 gram) eggplant, salted if necessary, cut into ½ inch cubes
- 1 medium onion, diced
- 5 garlic cloves, minced
- 1 (14 ounce or 400 gram) can diced tomatoes
- 1 cup canned crushed tomatoes
- 3 tablespoons capers
- 1 teaspoon crushed red pepper flakes, or to taste
- ½ teaspoon salt, plus more to taste
- ½ cup chopped fresh basil, plus more for serving, optional
- ¼ cup chopped fresh parsley, plus more for serving, optional
- Black pepper to taste

Instructions

1. Bring a large pot of salted water to a boil. Add the pasta and cook it according to the package directions, until al dente. Drain the pasta into a colander when it's finished cooking.

2. While the pasta cooks, coat the bottom of a large skillet with 2 tablespoons of olive oil and place it over medium heat. Once the oil is hot, add the diced eggplant in an even layer. (Notes 1 and 2)

3. Cook the eggplant for about 10 minutes, flipping the pieces only once or twice, until they're browned on multiple sides.

4. Remove the eggplant from the skillet and transfer it to a plate when it's finished browning.

5. While the eggplant cooks, coat the bottom of a large pot or skillet with the remaining 1 tablespoon of olive oil and place it over medium heat.

6. When the oil is hot, add the onion. Sweat the onion for about 5 minutes, until soft and translucent, stirring frequently.

7. Add the garlic and cook for 1 minute more, until very fragrant.

8. Stir in the diced tomatoes, crushed tomatoes, capers, red pepper flakes, and ½ teaspoon of salt.

9. Bring the sauce to a simmer, and allow it to cook, uncovered, for about 10 minutes, until it thickens up a bit. You can add a splash of water if it becomes too thick.

10. Stir the eggplant into the sauce and let the mixture simmer for about 5 minutes more, until the sauce very thick and the eggplant is very tender.

11. Add the cooked pasta, parsley and basil to the sauce and stir everything well to distribute the ingredients and wilt the herbs.

12. Remove the pot from heat and season the pasta with additional salt and black pepper to taste.

13. Divide onto plates and serve. Sprinkle with additional parsley and basil, if desired.

Prep Time: 15 Minutes

Cook Time: 10 Minutes

Servings: 4

Ingredients

- 10 ounces dried spaghetti
- 2 tablespoons olive oil
- 1 garlic clove, minced
- 1 tablespoon all-purpose flour
- ¾ cup full-fat coconut milk (from a can)
- 3 tablespoons lemon juice
- ½ teaspoon salt, plus more to taste (I use a full teaspoon, but that may be a lot for some folks.)
- 1 cup roughly chopped fresh basil
- ¼ teaspoon red pepper flakes, or to taste
- 1 tablespoon lemon zest
- Black pepper, to taste

Instructions

1. Bring a large pot of salted water to a boil and add the spaghetti. Cook it according to the package directions, then drain it into a colander.

Instructions

1. Add all ingredients except for the salt, pepper and hot sauce to a large (4 quart or larger) slow cooker.
2. Stir everything well to combine.
3. Cook the stew on high for 3 to 4 hours or low for 5 to 6 hours.
4. The stew is finished when the sauce is thick and the veggies are soft. At this point you can turn off the slow cooker, give it a stir, and season it with salt, pepper, and hot sauce to taste.
5. Ladle the stew into bowls and serve.